WOMB OF THE UNIVERSE

PREGNANCY: NUTRITION AND FITNESS

FIROZ TATA (WOLFY)

ISBN 978-1-63745-661-3

I would like to dedicate this work to the most precious lady Lord
Ahura Mazda could ever bestow on me and that is my adorable and
kindhearted mother, Ms. Heera Tata.

Your everloving son,

Firoz

Contents

Preface

It gives me immense bliss to bring my writing flair to the frontage by writing the book, 'Womb of the Universe'. I am confident that this publication of mine will gratify its purpose and will surely enrich the awareness among its readers to take perfect care before, during and after pregnancy; helping them to successfully navigate through the challenging nine months.

This book is prepared by keeping in mind the wearing and tough times expected mothers have to undergo. Love, care, compassion, sufficient rest along with nutrition and fitness are some of the dominant aspects of pregnancy. Inner peace, hygienic surrounding, staying stress-free and happy are some of the other important things that has to be taken care of during these decisive life-changing months. Most of the times pregnant women find themselves disheartened due to internal and external body changes. They feel exhausted, irritated and miserable because they fail to pay proper attention on their diet and fitness.

My book is all about nutrition and fitness that an expected mother has to look into. Changing the viewpoint in order to endeavour ahead towards happy, healthy and safe pregnancy is what my aim is behind creating this book. The book will assist its readers to understand nutritional and fitness value during and before being pregnant. After several hours of researching, collecting and scrutinizing various facts, the chapters are created in such a way that their reading, understanding and implementations on self will set you towards the path of happy pregnancy. After all, is is a beautiful feeling for parents to be able to relive their young days with the stunning 'little angle'? A mother brings priceless gift into the world. Therefore, truly a woman is considered as the 'Womb of the Universe'.

My book, 'Womb of the Universe' will assist you in enhancing and augmenting the knowledge towards creating a better pregnancy experience. Self-care and awareness towards pregnancy progress is all about having the right shift at the right time. This book has made an attempt to change the approach of the women towards overall concept of pregnancy for better health and future. I have no doubt that this book will be welcomed and appreciated equally by both who are pregnant or are planning to be.

Last but not least, I intend to inspire my loving readers to develop a positive mindset before and during pregnancy. The birth of a child does not doom the new mother to live a life with an untoned body, and thus, correct nutrition and fitness comes into a vital play. As always, I have tried my best to use reader-friendly, easy to understand and lucid language in the book. Let me assure you that this publication will not only go a very long way in easing the nine months of your pregnancy, but will also assist to discover and enjoy the divine blessing of pregnancy.

- **The Author**

Acknowledgements

From deep down my heart, I would like to express my sincere gratitude to my beloved mother Ms. Heera Tata to once again raise my spirit during the journey of writing this unexpected book as a single man and providing me with complete isolation while creating it. She has been a great support and helpful guide to me while writing this book.

I would also love to extend my heartfelt gratitude to Notion Press for providing a beautiful platform of Xpress Publishing, helping me to self-publish this ideal book, motivating my readers to pay more attention on their diet and fitness during and after pregnancy.

Last but not least, I also want to thank every single individual who says, "You have to buy this book" to their family members, friends and relatives.

- **The Author**

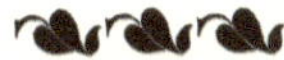

CHAPTER ONE

Introductory Words from the Heart

Getting pregnant and childbirth are two of the greatest miracles in woman's life. Many women often mention about pregnancy and childbirth when they are asked about the most memorable event in life. Birth of a child is like a precious gift from the heavens. There is just no denying about the powerful emotions that pregnancy and childbirth can create among parents; especially in the life of an expected mother.

While pregnancy is a splendid life changing and a rewarding experience, the hard truth is that there is a nutrition and fitness aspect too that cannot be ignored. Thus, there is a flip side to this shiny coin. Many women often end up feeling that pregnancy has ruined their attractive figure and the stretch marks have scarred them. They automatically start assuming that once they have given birth, their bodies will never go back to the shape they originally used to be. Weight gain, stretch marks, a loss of sex appeal, etc. are negative consequences that women consider a trade-off to have a baby.

Nothing could be further from the truth. Yes, pregnancy will result in weight gain. This is only natural and in fact, it's healthy. However, the gained weight can be maintained without letting it get out of control. All weight that is gained during pregnancy can be lost after pregnancy. After all, it's just fat and the principles of fat loss are same regardless if it's a pregnant woman or an obese man.

It may take time to shed the excess obesity, but there should not be any hurry as slow and steady wins the race. With patience and determination, a woman can definitely lose the excess fat after delivery. If a woman persists, she can even get fitter and be in a much better shape after childbirth than she had ever been. A human body is a marvellous structure and it can adapt to whatever demands we place upon it. The determination that it can be achieved is what truly matters. An untrue belief that pregnancy and childbirth will result in becoming a weighty, chubby or unpleasant woman must be completely released. The natural state of things will mean that a woman will gain weight during pregnancy and she will lose it all once the child is born.

- **Some of the important American female celebrities have had the following things to say about pregnancy and weight gain:**

(1) *"You have to eat to feed your baby. And I have a girl, so I want her to see some day why her mom has good self-esteem and good body issues. It gets you down sometimes, I'm not going to lie. I've had days where I'm like, 'Ugh, I wish this was easier.' But it's not, and that's OK."* - **Jennifer Love Hewitt** (an American actress, producer and singer)

(2) *"I am taking it week-by-week so I don't get frustrated with myself. If I had a long-term goal and that's all I thought about, I think it would set me back more."* - **Jessica Simpson**

(an American singer, actress, fashion designer and author)

(3) *"I think if you ask any pregnant mom, they're like 'I want my body back. But it takes time. It takes nine months for your body to get that way, and it's putting on that weight on purpose. The second I start to get down like, 'What happened to my body?' I look at my beautiful baby and I've never been more appreciative for this body that I have."* - **Hillary Duff** (an American producer, businesswoman and songwriter)

The point to learn from all this is that it is normal to gain weight and it takes time to lose it. A woman may feel down and depressed during this period. She can succeed in persisting and ultimately, she can get the body she had always desired.

There is much more to just losing weight after childbirth. She must be careful about her eating habits during pregnancy and how to do certain exercises to stay healthy, fit and strong. Therefore, this book will offer its readers some helpful tips and techniques that can be used to get healthy and stay in shape during and after the blessing of pregnancy.

CHAPTER TWO

The Stage of Preconception

Preconception care can be explained as a process aimed to identify and alter behavioural, biomedical and social risks to the woman's health or pregnancy outcome through preventive management. The goal of preconception care is to improve pregnancy outcomes and women's health in general through the prevention of ill health and diseases. It also manages the risk factors that affect pregnancy outcome and the health of future generation.

Before even getting pregnant, a woman should be aware that her health, habits, diet, fitness level and several other factors will directly or indirectly affect her pregnancy and the development of the fetus in her womb. For example: A pregnant woman with drinking or smoking habits can face serious complications for herself and her baby during pregnancy. Quitting all the undesirable and harmful habits prior to conception is what has to be understood by a to-be pregnant woman.

Ideally, she should exercise more, eat a clean diet, take sufficient sleep and surely avoid alcohol and smoking. If a woman has any issues with regard to substance abuse, she should eliminate it before planning to have a child.

Proper nutrition is crucial in the stages of preconception and during pregnancy. The beautiful baby in her womb is physically incapable to provide for itself. All the food and nutrition it gets is determined by the mother. The best for the baby and nothing less is what an expected mother must always try.

Initially, a fetus does not display any visible signs of malnourishment during the monthly check-ups. Thus, even the doctor will not be able to determine if the baby is getting all the necessary nutrients. A woman has to ensure that she is eating right and enough for the both. Getting all the needed vitamins and nutrients too is extremely essential for the growth of the baby. Only by being proactive and taking an active interest in nutrition, a woman will be able to keep both the baby and herself healthy and happy.

No one expects an unplanned pregnancy, but it happens often. In fact, about half of all pregnancies in the US are not planned. However, women can benefit from preconception health, whether or not they plan to have a baby one day. This is because part of preconception health is about people getting and staying healthy overall, throughout their lives. One of the best things a woman can do for herself is to take regular good care of her health. It is natural to think about eating various foods, but exercise too is an important aspect of staying healthy and fit.

- **Following are some of the important guidelines for preconception stage:**

(1) Mental health: Mental health is how we think, feel and act as we cope with various life challenges. To be at our best, one needs to feel good about life and should have self-value. Everyone feels concerned, apprehensive, depressed, sad or stressed sometimes, but pregnancy is a life changing experience. However, if you fail to get rid of such negative emotions and they keep on interfering in daily life, get help. Talk with your doctor or a health care professional about such feelings and treatment options.

(2) Smoking and alcohol: Smoking and consumption of alcohol for the expected mother is a big no. Smoking, drinking alcohol and using certain drugs can cause premature birth of the child, birth defects in child and even infant's death. If you are trying to get pregnant and cannot quit such habits, get help. Consult your doctor or visit a local medical centre.

(3) Helping partner: Asking the partner to play an active role during pregnancy is always beneficial. If your partner smokes or engages in damaging activities, they should immediately try and quit for the sake of the coming baby. If they fail to quit, they should not smoke around or tempt you by consuming alcohol around you.

(4) Health: Controlling health-related issues is essential. If a woman is asthmatic, obese, diabetic, etc. she should first get all these health related issues under control before getting pregnant. All these health problems may cause serious complications during pregnancy.

(5) Vaccinations: Certain important vaccinations are recommended before being pregnant, during pregnancy and right after the delivery. Having the right vaccination at the right time can avoid the mother and the baby from getting ill or having lifelong health problems.

(6) Staying fit: Getting fit and healthy, building strength and stamina makes pregnancy easy. Regular exercise is very important. During pregnancy, it becomes less taxing on the body if she is physically strong and healthy.

(7) Folic acid: There should be daily consumption of folic acid. Folic acid reduces the risk of birth defects related to the brain and spine. However, consulting the doctor about the same for an appropriate medical guidance is much needed.

(8) Toxic substances: Completely avoid harmful gases, synthetic chemicals, environmental pollutants and other toxic substances such as pesticides, fertilizer, metals, bug spray and dog or rodent feces around the home and in the workplace. These substances can harm the reproductive systems of both, men and women. They can make it more difficult to get pregnant. Exposure to even small amounts during pregnancy can lead to hazardous diseases.

CHAPTER THREE

Nutrition and Calories During Pregnancy

Hippocrates, also known as Hippocrates II, was an ancient Greek physician and one of the most outstanding figures in the history of medicine once quoted, *"Let food be thy medicine and let medicine be thy food."* This saying definitely holds true when one is pregnant. A clean, healthy and wholesome diet work wonders for a woman and her coming baby.

We live in a society that is overwhelmed with an excess of food choices. The harsh truth is that most of these foods are harmful to our body in the long run. In modern times, flavours, preservatives, colours, processed and junk foods, chemicals, genetically modified foods, etc. are all part of our regular diet. Gradually, they wreak havoc on human health.

Obesity and its relating health problems has become an epidemic, or one can even say a widespread pandemic. The number of people around the world suffering from diabetes, hypertension, high cholesterol, digestive disorders, etc. have risen steeply. The main culprit is the type of diet they consume. Changing one's diet and eating clean is an enormous task. It cannot be done overnight and even strong will-power sometimes fail to work. A person needs to make small gradual changes in the diet until clean eating habits are not developed. Thus, it is vital that such changes must be made at least three months before getting pregnant. Progressively, you will then be able to ease into a healthy diet relatively smoothly and easily.

Many women wonder about the amount of calories they need to consume during pregnancy. They hesitate to consume too many calories as they fear of putting on extra weight. Unfortunately, they have all these sudden food cravings that seemed to pop out of nowhere. However, do not get obsessed over your calories while pregnant because it is really not the time to analyse and count your calories. Fortunately, pregnancy gives you the consent to take nine months off from the calorie counting. That being said, it is also not a free pass to eat whatever food comes your way.

Eat sufficient, but eat the correct food. Restricting your calories could potentially harm your baby. Low birth weight, weakness in the mother, poor fetus development, etc. are often related to not consuming enough nutritious food during pregnancy. Whatever weight a mother gains can be burnt off after the childbirth. However, consuming over excess calories can result in bad health too. More than extra calories will gain too much weight that will put you at risk for diabetes, heart problems, early labour, pre-eclampsia, etc. Pre-eclampsia is a condition in which a pregnant woman develops high blood pressure. It can become very serious if not treated on time. Therefore, it is all about balancing. Eat enough for both yourself and your baby, but eat healthy and in moderation.

In the fitness industry, there is a saying, "Calories are not created equal." The saying tries to explain that if a person consumes 300 calories from two kinds of food, different results can be obtained. For example: If we eat two bananas and two apples a day, which would roughly be around 300 calories, what if we got all 300 calories from two scoops of ice cream? Would the benefits be the same? Which one is going to be better for the baby?

Good and healthy food choices are always beneficial irrespective of being pregnant or not. It doesn't matter if you are male or female, young or old; healthy diet in appropriate quantities is always helpful. The only difference is that now you are pregnant and it is even more important to eat right because another life too depends on you and is affected by your food choices.

- **Following are some of the types of food preferable during pregnancy:**

(1) Consuming whole foods: Whole foods are also known as single ingredient foods. For example, carrots are single ingredient food as they grow in the ground. On the other hand, let us take an example of white bread. Most of us have no idea how it is made, what ingredients are used and how do they get the bread so white. The moment you have no idea what goes into the food, it is best to avoid it. White bread is made from refined flour that is bleached white. Various artificial ingredients go into making a loaf. Such food stuffs will never do a pregnant body any favours. Avoiding processed foods and sticking to natural foods is what one needs to do.

(2) Consuming more vegetables and fruits: Vegetables and fruits contain an ocean of vitamins and minerals that are good for overall health. We all know, "An apple a day keeps the doctor away". Eating seven apples on one favourite day and expecting to get the job done is not sensible. It will never work that way as consistency with the diet is must.

(3) Consuming right kind of fats: Virgin coconut oil and olive oil are two of the best types of fats one can consume during pregnancy. Saturated fats are found in meat and dairy products such as ghee, butter and cheese. These foods too are best for the growth of the baby, if consumed in moderation.

(4) Consuming sufficient proteins: Proteins are an essential part of our daily diet. Protein can be obtained from lean meats, eggs, beef, beans, etc. Once again, focus on the single ingredient requirement. A few cuts of lean chicken breast are good. On the other hand, chicken nuggets are not good. Similarly, a slab of steak is good, but a few sausages are not healthy.

(5) Consuming good carbohydrates: Over the years, although carbohydrates have gained a bad reputation; the truth is that they too are essential for us. This is especially when one is pregnant. They give us energy and makes up a sizeable chunk of our required calories. However, it is essential to consume carbohydrates from healthy sources such as oats, fruits, brown rice, whole grain breads, vegetables, potatoes, quinoa, etc. Junk foods, white bread, white flour products, etc. have bad carbs that should be avoided even without being pregnant.

(6) Consuming organic foods: While this can be a little costly, it is highly beneficial. If you can afford and follow the practice of eating organic foods during the period of pregnancy, go for it. Organic foods are free of pesticides, growth regulators, synthetic fertilizers and livestock feed additives. Such foods are produced through farming practices that only use natural substances. The most commonly purchased organic foods are fruits, vegetables, meat, grains and dairy products. Nowadays, there are also many processed organic products available, such as sodas, cookies and breakfast cereals. If the budget doesn't permit to go completely organic, then make sure that at least some of the foods that you consume are organic. Unfortunately, some of the important foods such as apples, celery, cherries, bell peppers, grapes, pears, potatoes, raspberries, peaches, spinach and strawberries have been found to contain high levels of pesticides. Thus, sticking to organic products, is highly beneficial; especially during pregnancy.

- **Following are some of the essential vitamins available from various sources of food:**

(1) **Vitamin A:** eggs, carrots, mangoes, sweet potatoes, collard greens, cantaloupe, spinach and peas

(2) **Vitamin C:** bell peppers, citrus fruits, tomatoes, raspberries, green beans, strawberries, papaya, potatoes and broccoli

(3) **Vitamin D:** milk, fortified cereals, eggs and fatty fishes like salmon, catfish and mackerel

(4) **Vitamin E:** nuts, vegetable oil, wheat germ, spinach and fortified cereal

(5) **Vitamin B1:** pork, whole grains, eggs, wheat germ, and fortified cereals

(6) **Vitamin B2:** red meat, dairy products, pork, fish, whole grains, fortified cereals and eggs

(7) **Vitamin B3:** fish, eggs, meats, peanuts, whole grains, bread products, fortified cereals and milk

(8) **Vitamin B5:** mushrooms, meats, milk, eggs, peanuts and legumes

(9) **Vitamin B6:** bananas, baked potatoes, watermelon, fortified cereals, chicken breast and chickpeas

(10) Vitamin B7: cauliflower, chicken, mushroom and egg yolks

(11) Vitamin B8: legumes, seeds, eggs, cereals, green leafy vegetables and citrus fruits

(12) Vitamin B12: shellfish, red meat, fish, eggs and dairy products

(13) Calcium: spinach, dairy products, fortified butters and cereals, tofu, fortified juices, broccoli, sweet potatoes, lentils, okra, cabbage and kale.

(14) Iron: red meat, legumes, vegetables and grains

(15) Folic acid: strawberries, leafy vegetables, pasta, beetroots, peas, beans, broccoli, oranges and their juice, cauliflower, spinach, sunflower seeds and nuts

(16) Protein: yogurt, beans, poultry, protein bars, milk, red meat, fish, shellfish, eggs, cheese, tofu and fortified cereal

(17) Zinc: grains, red meats, nuts, oysters, poultry, beans, dairy products and fortified cereals

CHAPTER FOUR

Supplements Before and During Pregnancy

Besides food, a pregnant body also requires essential supplements. It is extremely difficult to get all the necessary nutrients, proteins, vitamins and minerals from the diet alone. Before and during pregnancy the diet has to be diverse and the knowledge of nutrition has to be good. This helps in getting a complete balanced diet with no deficiencies.

Most women do not have enough time to scrutinise their diet and note down the different nutrients they are getting through their diet. However, by consuming the prescribed supplements, it gets easy to compensate the loss from a diet that is deficient in a few vitamins and minerals. Therefore, some basic knowledge would be very helpful relating to what is being consumed, in what quantity and why that particular food is being consumed. This will help in getting pregnancy nutrition much safer, easier and correct.

One should be aware of the fact that there are negative consequences of overdosing of specific vitamins. This usually occurs by consuming diet that contains a certain vitamin and also consuming supplements simultaneously that contains same vitamin. This creates a surplus of same vitamin in the body. Therefore, it becomes important to tell your doctor during your prenatal appointments what kind of food you are eating and what medications and supplements you are consuming. This will help the doctor to assess your diet. Leaving out any details regardless of how insignificant you may consider them to be is not advisable.

- **Following are some of the important supplements that the doctor may prescribe during pregnancy:**

(1) Vitamin A: Vitamin A is crucial for the development of the baby's bones, heart, teeth, eyes, ears and immune system. Overdosing Vitamin A can cause birth defects and liver toxicity.

(2) Vitamin C: Vitamin C helps both, the mother and the baby to absorb iron. It even builds a healthy immune system. It also assists in holding the cells together and building the body tissues of the baby.

(3) Vitamin D: Vitamin D aids in the absorption of calcium. This will lead to healthy bones in the mother and the child. Babies usually require more Vitamin D than adults. As Vitamin D is rarely found in sufficient amounts in regular foods, usually doctors recommend its supplement. The formulation of the baby is fortified with the help of this vitamin. Vitamin D is also found in sunshine. Expected mothers having a mild deficiency of Vitamin D are advised to spend more time in the Sun.

(4) Vitamin E: Vitamin E helps in the formation of the child's body, muscles and red blood cells. It is better to get Vitamin E from natural food sources than synthetic supplements.

(5) Vitamin B1: It is also known as thiamine, assisting in the growth of child's organs and central nervous system.

(6) Vitamin B2: It is also known as riboflavin. It gives the body energy and helps in the development of the baby's bones, muscles and nervous system.

(7) Vitamin B3: It is also known as niacin. It helps to keep the mother's digestive system functioning optimally as well as gives the baby enough energy to develop well.

(8) Vitamin B6: It is also known as pyridoxine. It helps with the development of the baby's brain and nervous system. It also encourages the growth of new red blood cells in both, the mother and the child. Some pregnant women have claimed that Vitamin B6 has helped them to lessen their morning sickness.

(9) Vitamin B12: Vitamin B12 works together with folic acid to aid in the production of healthy red blood cells. It also promotes development of a healthy brain and nervous system in the baby. Usually, human body has sufficient stores of B12 and it is rare to have its deficiency.

(10) Protein: Protein is the building block of the body's cells. Protein is especially important in the second and third trimester when both, the mother and the baby are growing faster.

(11) Calcium: Calcium is vital for building the bones of the child. It also promotes the optimal functioning of the baby's heart and brain.

(12) Iron: This is yet another important vitamin that helps with cell development, placenta formation and blood cell formation.

(13) Zinc: It is necessary for the growth of the fetus. It aids in cell division and in the primary growth process of the baby's tiny tissues and organs. It also helps the mother and her baby to produce insulin and other enzymes.

(14) Folic acid: This is one of the most important vitamins essential during pregnancy. It is vital for the development of a healthy baby. Growth of the cells, replication of DNA and tissue formation is done with the help of this vitamin. Deficiency of folic acid may result in horrible birth defects such as spina bifida. Spina bifida is a medical condition in which some bones in the spinal cord are not developed normally at birth. Anencephaly, meaning underdevelopment of the brain is yet another nasty consequence. Such conditions occur during the first 28 days of conception. This is the period when usually the mother isn't aware of the fact that she is pregnant. Thus, it is essential that one gets enough folic acid through diet prior of getting pregnant.

CHAPTER FIVE

The Three Trimesters

Pregnancy can be divided into three trimesters. The first trimester starts from week 1 and ends at the 12th week. The second trimester begins from week 13 and ends at the 26th week. The third and final trimester commences from 27th week until the end of the pregnancy.

- **The First Trimester**

Nutrition: During the first trimester, calorie intake does not have to be significantly increased. However, one must ensure of getting all the right protein, vitamins, minerals, supplements if necessary, especially folic acid. This is not the period when the expected mother decides to do dieting or tries to keep her weight down. Enjoy the pregnancy process as it is normal to gain some pounds during the first trimester.

Exercise: Your strength and stamina prior to pregnancy determines how much exercise you can do during your first trimester. There is a misconception that pregnant women should not exercise for the fear of injuring their baby. This is not true. Pregnancy is not an excuse to become a couch potato. In fact, pregnancy gets easier if moderate activities are done regularly.

Avoiding high impact training regimens is always beneficial during the first trimester. One of the best forms of exercise that a pregnant woman can perform is brisk walking. In fact, just going for a daily 30-minute walk can work wonders. If you were highly active before pregnancy, for now you may miss your intense cardio sessions. However, you can still engage in cardio sessions as long as they are low in impact. A stationary bike is a good way to break a sweat.

Swimming during this phase of pregnancy too is an excellent form of exercise. Although it is a low impact exercise, yet very effective. High impact exercises such as skipping, full body workouts, kickboxing, etc. should be completely avoided.

Avoid strenuous workouts. Working out to the point where you feel breathless and gasping for air can prove dangerous. The aim must be to stay active and not train for some sports competition. Exercise helps to get the blood circulation right and normal functioning of the heart. Therefore, it is more about activity than achievement.

- **The Second Trimester**

Nutrition: The food choices will be the same for all the three trimesters. The only difference will be the amount of calories that will vary. As you step into your second and third trimester, the quantity of daily caloric intake increases. This helps to compensate for the increasing rate of your baby's growth. For example, if your pre-pregnancy caloric intake was 1500 calories, now it's time to consume 2100 calories a day. However, it is not the time to worry about the increasing weight. In fact, it is healthy to gain some weight during pregnancy. Eat correct foods and eat more so that there are sufficient calories and nutrients in your body for both you and your baby.

Exercise: Unlike the first trimester, most women do not experience morning sickness or fatigue during the second trimester. Gradually, the body adapts to the pregnancy. You may probably feel more energetic and active in your second trimester. Of course, in this trimester too the same rule applies about low impact exercises. However, now you should aim to incorporate strength training exercises in your regimen.

Paying more attention on exercises that tones back muscles, neck muscles and legs must be the aim of the expected mother. Pregnancy will create some strain on all these muscles. Often we hear from pregnant women complaining about their aching and tiring backs, necks and legs. Squats, lunges, bicep/triceps curls, modified side planks (knees at 90 degrees on ground), hip flexor, bird dog, step ups and straight leg calf stretch are some of the best strength exercises advised during the second trimester. As far as cardio goes, one may carry on with walking or stationary biking workout sessions.

Exercise depends from individual to individual. There are women who are extremely sporty before pregnancy and can go running or even play certain sports during pregnancy. This totally depends on person's stamina and capabilities. Your doctor is the best person who can advise you on various types of exercises that will suite you depending on your condition.

Generally, most women prefer walking or doing a stationary biking. There is really no need to overdo it or try and prove that pregnancy is not holding you back. Do not exercise more than your limits just because you are consuming more calories during your second trimester and you want to burn them off to stay slim. This will affect you and the baby adversely.

Enjoy pregnancy as a blessing and keep spreading a happy glow of being a pregnant woman.

- **The Third Trimester**

Nutrition: By now, you must have had undergone several appointments with your doctor, to monitor your pregnancy progress. The calorie requirement in the third trimester will be determined by your condition. The doctor will advise you if you need to eat more or less. Just follow his/her instructions.

Exercise: By now, the baby bump will be seen significantly. It may hinder most of the exercise and movements that you are accustomed to. However, you will still be able to go for walking or use a stationary bike. The goal is just to stay moving. Do not focus on sweating or getting the heart rate up. It is not about intensity but about mobility. Meditate and relax to clear your mind and feel stress-free. There is immense power in mediation. Alternatively, you can join a few classes of yoga specifically designed for pregnant women. These classes often focus on stretching and also release the tension in the back, legs and neck area.

In the final trimester, every movement might be a challenging effort. If you feel like you are not in a mood to exercise or it is just too much effort, take a break. Being happy matters a lot during pregnancy because if the mother stays happy, the baby will be happy too.

CHAPTER SIX

Body Shaping After Pregnancy

This is the part where you cuddle your new-born and make cooing noises. It is the phase where if you are fortunate enough you can order your partner to fulfil your every request because you are on the path of recovery. After childbirth, you can slowly reduce your calorie consumption. Carry on with your clean eating habits. As you will be lactating and will need to breastfeed your infant, eat nutritious food in sufficient quantities. Once again, the best person to consult to, will be your doctor.

Lack of knowledge, poor family and social support, social norms, awkwardness, child care, lactation problems, employment and child care, etc. are some of the barriers to breastfeeding. Generally, there are a few breastfeeding ways that the new mother should be aware of. As breastfeeding may hurt, moisturizing the area with olive oil can help. Drinking ample amount of water to stay hydrated at all the time further helps. Eating well and consuming adequate amount of calories is essential. A new mother can learn all these and various other things relating to nursing her child from numerous sources. A good guide book for new mothers is one of them.

Getting the body back in its shape after childbirth is necessary for the mother's good health. After couple of weeks or little more, you can get ready to start on with your exercise program. Start shedding the excess weight. Once again you will check your daily caloric requirement. As soon as you have a number, you will aim for a particular amount of calorie deficit daily. Do not aim cutting the calories too low. This won't speed up your results. It will just plateau your body and obstruct any further progress.

Now that you have given birth to a child, you can exercise often. However, there are a few things you must be aware of. It takes six to twelve weeks for the body to heal after pregnancy. This means still you should follow a training program that is low in intensity. Although low impact training will be your mantra, still you will succeed in losing the excess weight at a steady rate. As long as your body is at a caloric deficit, you will lose weight. If you walk twice a day with each session lasting 30 to 45 minutes, you will be amazed to see how much weight you will lose.

As long as your diet is clean and healthy and you are at a daily caloric deficit you will lose weight. Many women get impatient and expects fast results. Weight loss is not an overnight process. It does not matter if you are pregnant or not. Losing weight is a taxing task that takes time, hard work and determination. Never give up on it just because you think it will take another nine months to lose all the gained weight. You will still be where you are if you do not make an active effort to change yourself. Most women can return to their pre-pregnancy body shape within six months, just by doing low impact cardio daily and maintaining a caloric deficit. If they can do it, so can you.

CHAPTER SEVEN

Taking Fitness to the Next Level

It is recommended to visit the doctor after a few months and check if you are able to increase the intensity of your training program. Once you get the consent, it is time to work little hard over your body. Start training with weights and combine your resistance training with cardio sessions. Keep your cardio sessions short but at a high-intensity. This will put your body in a fat burning mode for hours. The principles are the same, a caloric deficit and training. Thus, to shift yourself from moderately fit to super fit is just a matter of gradual intensity and time.

The more intensely you train the better your results will be. Train passionately for two to three months and that will work wonders on your body. Spending a year in training will be awesome. The longer the duration, the better your body will transform.

Mindset too plays a significant role. The birth of a newborn does not doom the new mother to live life with an untoned body. It is not a lifelong curse of being obese. In fact, there is nothing stopping you from getting the desired body. The only thing that stops you is your own self.

You are a mother and you have every reason to be a living example for your child. Set a fitness goal for yourself. Endeavour towards it. Stay focused and set small quantifiable aims. Be happy with the small feats and cherish them. The end goal is a result of all the milestones you reached along the way. Before you realise, you will have the body your heart desires.

People often put others down to lift themselves up. It helps them see past their own failings and fulfil their egos. However, only you are aware that it took efforts, discipline and determination to transform for the good. Aren't these the qualities you want your child to possess? Of course, you do. Children learn more by watching what elders do rather than by listening to what they say. Be the best example for your child as it is truly priceless. Feeling fat lasts only for a few months, but the joy and blessing of being a mother lasts always and forever.

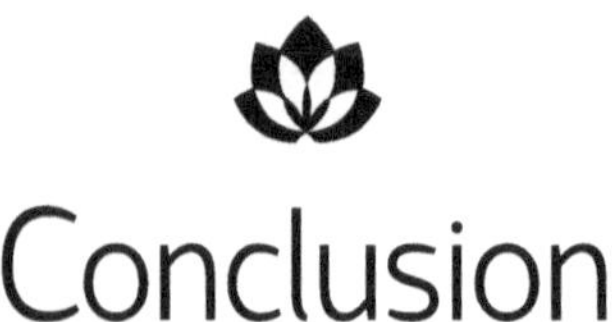

CHAPTER EIGHT

Conclusion

When a baby girl is born, with the correct amount of love, care, respect, dignity, discipline and compassion she grows into a beautiful woman of substance and strength. As the natural cycle keeps progressing, she grows old enough and becomes a mother, nurturing a life within herself and beyond. She develops a new life and creates a whole new world within her womb. It's magical and miraculous.

She is the lady of the house, doing her tasks with utmost care, love and sympathy. She fails at times, yet ready for another challenge. She is a daughter; parent's most prized jewel, a sister; the one she grows up with disagreeing most of the times yet the most protective one, a lover; desiring for respect and warmth, a selfless partner; being that one steady rock who understands without efforts, a wife; choosing family over herself every day and a mother; the unconditional source of pure love, care and nurturing.

Ask a father how blessed a man he is if he gets to nurture the nurturer. Ask a mother, how beautiful it would be for her to be able to relive her young days with the graced one she has brought into the world. Truly a woman is considered as the 'Womb of the Universe'.

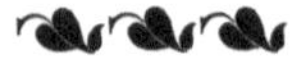

www.ingramcontent.com/pod-product-compliance
Lightning Source LLC
Chambersburg PA
CBHW031435250726